A. Sri Sennath J. Arul
Sonika Verma
A. Sri Sennath J. Arul

Genetic Disorders

A. Sri Kennath J. Arul
Sonika Verma
A. Sri Sennath J. Arul

Genetic Disorders

A Brief Review

LAP LAMBERT Academic Publishing

Impressum / Imprint

Bibliografische Information der Deutschen Nationalbibliothek: Die Deutsche Nationalbibliothek verzeichnet diese Publikation in der Deutschen Nationalbibliografie; detaillierte bibliografische Daten sind im Internet über http://dnb.d-nb.de abrufbar.
Alle in diesem Buch genannten Marken und Produktnamen unterliegen warenzeichen-, marken- oder patentrechtlichem Schutz bzw. sind Warenzeichen oder eingetragene Warenzeichen der jeweiligen Inhaber. Die Wiedergabe von Marken, Produktnamen, Gebrauchsnamen, Handelsnamen, Warenbezeichnungen u.s.w. in diesem Werk berechtigt auch ohne besondere Kennzeichnung nicht zu der Annahme, dass solche Namen im Sinne der Warenzeichen- und Markenschutzgesetzgebung als frei zu betrachten wären und daher von jedermann benutzt werden dürften.

Bibliographic information published by the Deutsche Nationalbibliothek: The Deutsche Nationalbibliothek lists this publication in the Deutsche Nationalbibliografie; detailed bibliographic data are available in the Internet at http://dnb.d-nb.de.
Any brand names and product names mentioned in this book are subject to trademark, brand or patent protection and are trademarks or registered trademarks of their respective holders. The use of brand names, product names, common names, trade names, product descriptions etc. even without a particular marking in this works is in no way to be construed to mean that such names may be regarded as unrestricted in respect of trademark and brand protection legislation and could thus be used by anyone.

Coverbild / Cover image: www.ingimage.com

Verlag / Publisher:
LAP LAMBERT Academic Publishing
ist ein Imprint der / is a trademark of
AV Akademikerverlag GmbH & Co. KG
Heinrich-Böcking-Str. 6-8, 66121 Saarbrücken, Deutschland / Germany
Email: info@lap-publishing.com

Herstellung: siehe letzte Seite /
Printed at: see last page
ISBN: 978-3-659-35495-3

CONTENTS   **Page No.**

I. INTRODUCTION

Genetic Disorders: A pathological condition caused by an absent o defective gene or by a chromosomal aberration. Also called hereditary disease or inherited disorder.

Or it is a disease that is caused by an abnormality in an individual's DNA. Abnormalities can range from a small mutation in a single gene to the addition or subtraction of an entire chromosome or set of chromosomes.

Genetic disorders are far more common than is widely appreciated. The lifetime frequency of genetic diseases is estimated to be 670/1000. The genetic diseases encountered in medical practice represent only the tip of iceberg that is those with less extreme genotype errors permitting full embryonic development and live birth. It is estimated that 50% of spontaneous abortuses during the early months of gestation have a demonstrable chromosomal abnormality; there are, in addition, numerous small detectable errors and many others still beyond our range of identification. About 1% of all newborn infants possess a gross chromosomal abnormality, and approximately 5% of individuals under 25 develop a serious disease with a significant genetic component.

II. TYPES OF GENETIC DISORDERS:

These are the diverse group of disorders that can be considered under the following headings:

1. *Single-gene disorders* caused by the presence of a single muted gene that result in the synthesis of a defective protein. Mutations may be inherited or arise de-novo in the parent's germ cells.

2. *Chromosomal aberrations* that involves loss or gain of chromosomes, alteration in the chromosome structure and different chromosome constitutions in two or more cell lines.

3. *Multifactorial disorders* caused by the complex interactions between genes and environmental factors.

4. Still other genetic disorders are caused by *mutations in mitochondrial DNA*.

1. SINGLE-GENE DISORDERS

These are a group of diseases caused by the presence of a single muted gene. The mutation alters the coding information of the gene such that it either produces defective protein or fails to produce any protein at all. The resulting protein deficiency is responsible for the disease symptoms.

Mutations that caused single gene disorders are diverse. Broadly they are of two types: *point mutations* that involve single base changes and *gross mutations* that involve large DNA sequences.

For each disorder, the type of mutation presently varies. In addition, individuals affected by the same disorders may carry different mutations. A number of different types of point mutations exist. These are missence mutations, non-sense mutations, frameshift mutations, splice site mutations and promoter mutations. Gross mutations include deletions, insertions, and rearrangements.

The gene mutation may be passed between generations from parents to children or may arise spontaneously in a germ cell of a parent or de-novo. Three pattern of inheritance occur: *autosomal dominant, autosomal recessive and X-linked.*

3

Autosomal Dominant Inheritance:

In Autosomal Dominant Inheritance, the following characteristics should be observed:

1. Every affected person has at least one affected parent.

2. Males and females are likely to be affected equally and should be capable of transmitting the trait, provided the affected gene does not cause sterility.

3. Usually there is no skipping of generations, and father-to-son and mother-to-daughter transmission should be as frequent as father-to-daughter and mother-to-son.

4. Affected persons typically transmit the trait to half of their offspring.

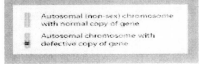

Examples of diseases exhibiting autosomal dominant inheritance are *Achondroplasia, Neurofibromatosis, Osteogenesis imperfecta, Dentinogenesis imperfecta, Dentine dysplasia, some forms of amelogenesis imperfecta, Epidermolysis bullosa simplex, Marfan syndrome, Naevoid basal cell carcinoma syndrome.*

Autosomal Recessive Inheritance:

This trait makes up the largest category of Mendelian disorders. Because autosomal recessive disorders result only when both alleles at a given gene loci are mutated; such disorders are characterized by the following features:

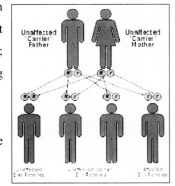

The following characteristics should be observed:

1. The trait does not usually affect the parents of the affected individual, but siblings may show the disease.

2. Siblings have one chance in four of having the trait.

4

3. If the mutant gene occurs with low frequency in the population, there is strong likelihood that the affected individual (proband) is the product of consanguineous marriage.

Examples are: *Epidermolysis bullosa (Junctional and Dystrophic type), Sickle cell disease, Thalassemia, Ehler-Danlos syndrome (some variants).*

X-Linked Recessive Inheritance:

The transmission of X-chromosomes from parents to offspring provides the basis for the pattern of X-linked (sex-linked) recessive inheritance. Affected males cannot transmit an X-linked gene to their sons since sons receive the Y-chromosome; but all daughters will receive the gene and be carriers. Father-to-son transmission of a trait rules out X-linked genes.

Criteria for X-linked recessive inheritance:

1. Incidence of the trait is much higher in males than in females.

2. The trait is transmitted by affected men to all of their daughters, who are carriers.

3. The trait cannot be transmitted from father to son.

4. The trait may be transmitted through a series of carrier females, and if so the affected males in a family are related to one another through these carrier females.

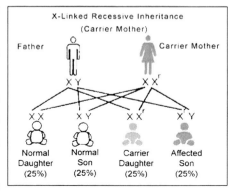

Some diseases of dental importance which are transmitted by genes on the X- chromosome are *Anhidrotic ectodermal dysplasia and Hemophilia A and B, Chronic granulomatous disease.*

X-Linked Dominant Inheritance:

The rules for X-linked dominant inheritance are similar to those for X-linked recessive, except that in the former heterozygous females may express the condition.

Since females have twice as many X-chromosomes as males, they exhibit a higher frequency of the trait. An affected female, if heterozygous, will transmit the gene to one-half other offspring, regardless of their sex.

However, an affected male cannot transmit the trait to his sons, but all his daughters receive his X-chromosome containing the affected gene and hence will be affected.

Examples are: *Vitamin D resistant rickets (hypophosphatemia), Oro-facial-digital syndrome, and amelogenesis imperfecta (hypoplastic type).*

Y-Linked (Holandric) Inheritance:

It implies that only males are affected. An affected male transmits Y-linked traits to all of his sons but to none of his daughters. In the past, it has been suggested that bizarre-sounding conditions such as porcupine skin, hairy ears and webbed toes are Y-linked traits.

With the possible exception of hairy ears, these claims of holandric inheritance have not stood up to more careful study.

Evidence clearly indicates, however, that the H-Y histocompatibility antigen and genes involved in spermatogenesis are carried on the Y-chromosome and, therefore, manifest holandric

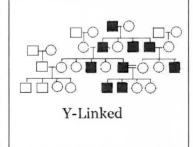

Y-Linked

inheritance. The latter, if deleted, leads to infertility from azoospermia.

To date, over 10,000 single gene disorders have been identified in humans. Most are rare but together they affect 1-2 % of the population at any one time.

The following are some of the more important and common single gene disorders.

➤   *Huntington's disease (HD)*: It is an **autosomal dominant** disorder, which affects about 1 in 10,000 people. A person usually does not experience symptoms until they are at least 30 to 40 years old. At that time, or even later in life, a person with Huntington's disease develops uncontrolled movements called chorea and may also have problems with coordination, thinking, and judgment. These symptoms are due to the degeneration of nerve cells in a part of the brain called the basal ganglia in the cerebrum. This degeneration typically progresses until it results in the person's death. Intellectual changes in the early stages of HD include memory impairment and poor concentration span. Anxiety and panic attacks, mood changes, depression, aggressive behavior, paranoia, increased libido and alcohol abuse can also occur.

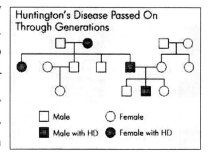

The defective gene responsible for HD is called **huntingtin** and is mapped on chromosome 4. The gene is expressed in many cells in CNS but the function of its encoded protein is unclear. Recent evidence suggests a possible role in apoptosis. The nature of the defect in gene causing HD is unusual. The gene contains a repeated CAG sequence near the 5'end. In normal individuals, the sequence is repeated 26 times or less. But in HD the repeat sequence is expanded and occurs more than 40 times. The size of HD expansion correlates inversely with age at onset. Greater instability of expansion is observed with paternal HD and juvenile onset in offspring.

➤   *Duchenne muscular dystrophy (DMD):* It is an **X-linked recessive** disorder and affected males suffer progressive weakening of the muscles. It affects 1:3500 males. Symptoms first appear in the age of 3 to 5 years with slow progressive muscle weakening resulting in awkward gait, inability to run quickly, difficulty in rising from floor. Subsequent deterioration occurs leads to lumber lordosis, joint contractures and cardio-respiratory failure; resulting in death at the mean age of 18 years.

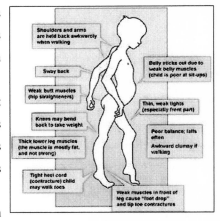

On examination, boys show an apparent increase in the size of calf muscles; this is actually due to replacement of muscle fibres by fat and connective tissue, referred to as pseudohypertrophy.

The gene responsible for DMD is present on the X-chromosome. About two-thirds of mutations found in DMD patients are deletions. The size and the location of the deletions vary but the two regions of the DMD gene, one involving the first 20 exons and the second near the centre of the gene are affected more often. Mutations identified in the remaining one-third cases of DMD patients are point mutations which results in reduced or absent gene expression. These include non-sense, frameshift, splicing and promoter mutations.

The DMD gene encodes a large protein called *dystrophin*, which has a structural role in muscle cells and absence of such protein causes gradual degeneration of muscle cells. Gene therapy offers the only realistic hope of a future cure of DMD.

➢ *Cystic fibrosis (CF)*: It is an *autosomal recessive* single-gene disorder is that was first recognized as a discrete entity in 1936 and used to be known as 'mucoviscidosis' because of the accumulation of thick mucus secretion that lead to blockage of the airway and secondary infection. CF is one of the most common autosomal recessive disorders encountered in individuals of Western European origin, in whom the incidence varies from 1:2000 to 1:3000.

The organs most commonly affected in CF are the lungs and the pancreas. Chronic lung disease caused by recurrent infection eventually leads to fibrotic changes in the lungs with secondary cardiac failure, a condition known as Cor-pulmonale. When this complication occurs, the only hope for long term survival rests in a successful heart –lung transplant. In 85% of individuals with CF, pancreatic function is impaired, leading to malabsorption. Other problems include nasal polyps, rectal prolapsed, cirrhosis and diabetes mellitus.

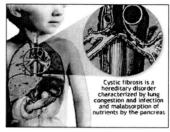

Cystic fibrosis is a hereditary disorder characterized by lung congestion and infection and malabsorption of nutrients by the pancreas

The defective gene in CF is the **CFTR gene** locus mapped to chromosome 7q31. This encodes a large cell membrane protein which acts as a chloride channel. The CFTR protein removes chloride ions from cells and alters the sodium chloride balance, thus reducing the viscosity of mucus secretion. The inevitable fatal outcome in CF and the current lack of an effective treatment have led to attempts to develop a cure based on gene therapy.

➢ *Marfan syndrome (MFS):* It is a disorder of fibrous connective tissue that follows ***autosomal dominant*** inheritance. Affected individuals are tall, have joint laxity, a reduced upper to lower segment body ratio, pectus deformity and scoliosis.
The connective tissue defect gives rise to ectopia lentis and dilatation of ascending aorta.
The majority of cases are linked to the large ***FBN1 gene*** on 15q21, with 65 exons spanning 200kb and containing five distinct domains. The gene encodes for type I fibrillin, a glycoprotein. Most mutations are missence and have a dominant-negative effect resulting in less than 35% of the expected amount of fibrillin in the extracellular matrix.

➢ *Neurofibromatosis (NF):* This is one of the most common genetic disorders in humans and gained public notoriety then it was suggested that Joseph Merrick, the 'Elephant Man' was probably affected. There are two main types NF1 and NF2 having birth incidence of 1:3000 and 1:35000 respectively. The most notable features of NF1 are café-au-lait spots and neurofibromas. Other 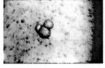 findings include relative macrocephaly and Lisch nodules.

NF1 shows *autosomal dominant* inheritance with virtually 100% penetrance at the age of 5 years. Approximately 50% cases of NF1 are due to new mutations or it can be the result of gonadal mosaicism (usually paternal in origin) as seen in the affected child born to unaffected parents. The NF1 gene, *neurofibromin*, is mapped to chromosomes 17 adjacent to the centromere. The neurofibromin protein encoded by this gene shows structural homology to the guanosine triphosphatase activation protein (GAP), and acts as a tumor suppressor protein, which is important in signal transduction. Other genes including TP53 and the short arm of chromosome 17 are also involved in tumor development and progression of NF 1.

Conversely, neurofibromin gene is implicated in the development of sporadic tumors not associated with NF, including colon carcinoma, neuroblastoma and malignant melanoma. These observations confirm that neurofibromin gene plays an important role in cell growth and differentiation.

Many different mutations have been identified in neurofibromin gene which includes deletions, insertions, duplications and point substitutions leading to severe truncation of the protein or complete absence of the gene expression.

At present there is no cure for NF 1. Drug therapy aim at upregulating neurofibromin GAP activating or down regulating RAS activity could prove beneficial in the absence of effective gene therapy.

➢ *Tay-Sach's Disease:* It is a well known sphingolipidosis with an incidence of 1:3600 in Ashkenazi Jews and follows *autosomal recessive* inheritance. Infants usually present by 6 months of age with poor feeding, lethargy and floppiness. Developmental regression usually becomes apparent in late infancy; feeding becomes increasingly difficult, and the infant progressively deteriorates with deafness, visual impairment and spasticity, which progresses to rigidity. Death usually occurs by the age of 3years from respiratory infection. Less severe juvenile, adult, and chronic forms are reported.

The diagnosis is supported clinically by the presence of a cherry-red spot in the centre of macula of the fundus. Biochemical confirmation of Tay-Sach's disease is by demonstration of reduced *hexosaminidase A* levels in serum, white blood cells or cultured fibroblasts, and direct gene analysis is available. Reduced hexosaminidase A activity is due to deficiency of the subunit of the enzyme ß-hexosaminidase, that leads to accumulation of the sphingolipid GM_2 ganglioside.

➢   Some single-gene disorders are not entirely dominant or entirely recessive. In these disorders, each member of a pair of genes has a distinct effect. This is sometimes referred to as *co-dominant, semi-dominant, or intermediate expression*. An example of such a disorder is *sickle-cell anemia* It is the most common hemoglobinopathy caused by point mutation resulting in substitution of glutamine with valine at codon 6 of the β globin polypeptide. The mutation is therefore a single base-pair in the triplet code at this point, from GAC to GTC.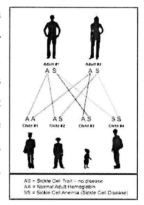

The abnormal hemoglobin produced is HbS. Such substitution makes HbS less soluble than normal Hb and causes HbS molecules to polymerize. This distorts the shape of red blood cells under deoxygenated conditions, so called sickling. The clinical manifestations are manifold and include painful sickle cell crisis, chest crisis, aplastic crisis, splenic sequestration crisis, retinal disease, cerebrovascular accident. Sickled cells with distorted cell membranes are taken up by the reticuloendothelial system. The shorter red cell survival time leads to a more rapid red cell turnover and consequently anemia.

The heterozygous or carrier state for the SC allele is known as *sickle cell trait* and is generally not associated with any significant health risk.

➤ A category of single-gene disorders known as X-linked disorders involves genes located on the X chromosome, one of the two sex chromosomes. Males are at greater risk for X-linked genetic disorders than females, because if a male inherits an X chromosome with a mutated recessive gene, he lacks a second X chromosome that might provide the normal, dominant form of the gene. The Y chromosome contains only a small number of genes that are mostly involved in determining male characteristics. Alterations to genes on the Y chromosome are a factor in some instances of male infertility. An example of an *X-linked recessive* disorder is *Hemophilia*. It is of two types: Hemophilia A and Hemophilia B.

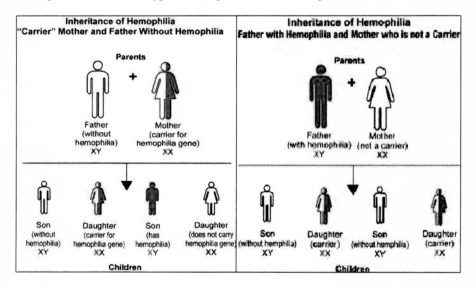

Hemophilia A is the most common severe inherited coagulation disorder with an incidence of 1:5000 males; caused by deficiency of factor VIII, which along with factor IX, plays a critical role in intrinsic coagulation pathway. Hemophilia B affects 1:40,000 males and is caused by deficiency of factor IX. The clinical features may vary from mild bleeding following major trauma or surgery to spontaneous hemorrhage into muscles and joints. The degree of similarity shows a close correlation with the reduction in factor VIII or IX activity.

Both forms of hemophilia show X-linked recessive inheritance. The loci lie close together near the distal end of Xq. The factor VIII comprises 26 exons and spans 186 kb with a 9-kb mRNA transcript. Deletions account for 5% of all cases and usually cause complete absence of factor VIII expression. In addition, frameshift, nonsense and missense mutations have been described, besides insertions and flick inversions. Point mutations usually originate in male germ cells where as deletion arise mainly in female. Factor IX gene comprised 8 exons is a 34-kb long. More than 800 different point mutations, deletions and insertions have been reported.

Hemophilia A and B are excellent candidate for gene therapy as only a slight increase in the plasma level of the relevant factor is of major clinical benefit.

The examples of other single-gene disorders are:
✓   Myotonic dystrophy
✓   Hereditary motor and sensory neuropathy
✓   Loeys- Dietz Syndrome
✓   Congenital contractural arachnodactyly
✓   Inherited cardiac arrhythmias and cardiomyopathies
✓   Spinal muscular atrophy

2. CHROMOSOMAL ABERRATIONS

Chromosomal aberrations can either be due to alteration in the structure of chromosomes (Structural abnormalities) or alteration in number of chromosomes (Numerical aberrations) or different chromosome constitutions in two or more cell lines (Mixoploidy).

A.   Structural Abnormalities:

1. **Deletion**: It involves loss of a part of a chromosome. It is of two types: a) **Terminal deletion**: It involves single break and the terminal part of the chromosome is lost. E.g. *Wolf-Hirschhorn and Cri-du-chat syndrome*, which involves loss of material from the short arms of chromosomes 4 and 5 respectively. In both conditions

severe learning difficulties is usual, often with failure to thrive. Cri-du-chat syndrome derives its name from the characteristic cat like cry of affected neonates; a consequence of underdevelopment of larynx. Both conditions are rare with estimated incidences of approximately 1:50,000 births.

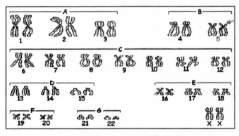

Cri-du-chat syndrome karyotype

b) *Interstitial deletion*: It involves two breaks and the intervening portion of the chromosome is lost e.g. *Prader-Willi syndrome (PWS)* characterized by short stature, obesity, hypogonadism and learning difficulty. Approximately 50%-60% of individuals with PWS can be shown to have an interstitial deletion of proximal portion of the long arm of chromosome 15. DNA analysis has revealed that the chromosome deleted is almost always the paternally derived homolog. Remaining 25%-30% of individuals with PWS, without a chromosomes deletion, have been shown to have maternal uniparental disomy.

Another example of interstitial deletion is *Wilm's tumor*. It is a rare renal embryonal neoplasm. Children with Wilm's tumor also have aniridia, genitourinary abnormalities and retardation of growth and development. This combination is referred to as WAGR syndrome. Chromosomal analysis reveals an interstitial deletion of 11p13. The deletion gene includes PAX6, responsible for aniridia.

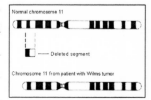

2.   **Duplication**: Duplications of chromosomal segments can occur by the breakage-fusion-bridge cycle or by crossovers within the loop of an inversion.

3.   **Insertions**: An insertion occurs when a segment of one chromosome becomes inserted into another chromosome. If the inserted material has moved from elsewhere in another chromosome, then the karotype is balanced. Otherwise an

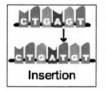

Insertion

14

insertion causes an unbalanced chromosome complement. Carriers of a balanced deletion-insertion re-arrangement are at a 50% risk of producing unbalanced gametes, as random chromosome segregation at meiosis will result in 50% of the gametes inheriting either the deletion or the insertion, but not both.

4.   **Inversion:** Two breaks in the same chromosomes can lead to inversion, in which middle section is reattached but in the inverted configuration. Crossing over with inversion loops results in semi-sterility. Almost all gametes that contain dicentric or imbalanced chromosomes form inviable zygote. Thus a certain proportion of the progeny of inversion heterozygotes are not viable.

If the inversion segment involves the centromere, it is termed as ***pericentric inversion***). If it involves only one arm of chromosome, it is termed as ***paracentric inversion***.

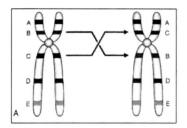 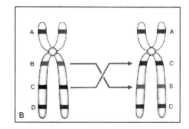

5.   **Translocation:** Breaks can occur simultaneously in two non-homologous chromosomes. There are various ways in which reunion can occur. The most interesting case occurs when the ends of two non-homologous chromosomes are translocated to each other, which is called ***reciprocal translocation***. The organism, in which this has happened, a reciprocal translocation heterozygote, has all the genetic

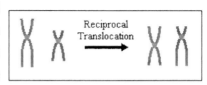

material of the normal homozygote. Two outcomes of a reciprocal translocation are new linkage arrangements in a homozygote organism with translocated chromosomes only and variegation position effects.

One such example of reciprocal translocation is *chronic myeloid leukemia*. In 1960, investigators in Philadelphia were the first to describe an abnormal chromosome in white blood cells from patients with chronic myeloid leukemia (CML). The abnormal chromosome, referred to as *Philadelphia chromosome (Ph¹)*, is an acquired abnormality found in blood or bone marrow cells but not in other tissues

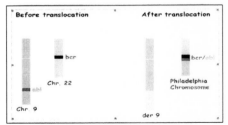

from these patients. The Ph¹ is a tiny chromosome that is now known to be a chromosome 22 from which long arm material has been reciprocally translocated to and from the long arm of chromosome 9 i.e. *t (9;22)* (q34;q11). This chromosomal re-arrangement is seen in 90% of those with CML.

The second type is **Robertsonian translocation** that is a particular type of reciprocal translocation in which the breakpoints are located at, or close to the centromeres of two acrocentric chromosomes. This is also referred as *centric fusion*. The short arms of each chromosomes are lost, this being of no clinical importance as they contain genes only for ribosomal RNA, for which there are

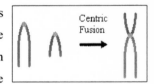

multiple copies on the various other acrocentric chromosomes. The total chromosome number is reduced to 45. As there is no loss or gain of important genetic material, this is a functionally balanced re-arrangement.

The major practical importance of Robertsonian translocation is that they can predispose to the birth of babies with *Down syndrome*; as a result of embryo inheriting two normal number 21 chromosomes, plus a translocation chromosome involving a number 21 chromosome. The clinical consequences are exactly the same as those seen in typical trisomy 21; the parent of child with translocation Down syndrome has a relatively high risk of having further affected children if one of them carries the re-arrangement in the balanced form.

6.   **Ring chromosomes:** A ring chromosome is formed when a break occurs on each arm of the chromosome leaving two sticky ends on the central portion that re-

unite as a ring. The two distal chromosomal fragments are lost so that, if the involved chromosome is an autosome, the effects are usually serious. Ring chromosomes are often unstable in mitosis so that it is common to find a ring chromosome in only a proportion

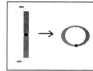

of cells. The other cells in the individual are usually monosomic because of the absence of the ring chromosome.

7.   **Iso-chromosomes:** An isochromosome shows loss of one arm with duplication of the other. The most probable explanation for the formation of an isochromosome is that the centromere has divided transversely rather than longitudinally. The most commonly encountered isochromosome is that which consists of two long arms of X-chromosome. This accounts for up to 15% of all cases of Turner's syndrome.

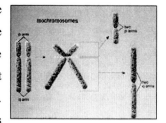

B. Numerical Abnormalities:

Changes in chromosome number are of two basic types: changes in whole chromosome sets called aberrant euploidy and changes in part of chromosome sets, resulting in aneuploidy.

1.   **Aberrant Euploidy**: Organisms that have more or less than the normal number of sets are aberrant euploids. Polyploids are individual organisms in which there are more than two chromosome sets. They can be represented by 3n (triploid), 4n (tetraploid).

Polyploidy: Polyploid cells contain multiples of the haploid number of chromosomes such as 69, triploidy or 92, tetraploidy. Triploidy is caused by failure of a maturation meiotic division in an ovum or sperm, leading to retention of a barr body or to the formation of a diploid sperm. Alternatively, it can be caused by fertilization of an ovum by two sperms: known as dispermy. Triploidy (69,XXX; 69,XXY; 69,XYY) is a relatively common finding in material cultured from spontaneous abortions, but is seen rarely in a live born infant. Child shows severe intrauterine growth retardation with relative preservation of head growth at the expense of a small thin trunk. Syndactyly involving the third and fourth fingers and/or the second and third toes is a common finding.

2. Aneuploidy: It is the second major category of chromosomal aberrations. An aneuploid is an individual organism, whose chromosome number differs from the wild type by a part of a chromosome set. Aneuploid nomenclature is based on the number of copies of the specific chromosome in the aneuploid state. The aneuploid condition 2n-1 is called monosomy and 2n+1 is called trisomy.

a) Monosomy: The absence of a single chromosome is referred to as monosomy. It results from non-disjunction in meiosis. Lack of contribution of an X or Y chromosome results in a *45, X karyotype*, causing the condition called as *Turner's syndrome*. It affects one in ten thousand live female births. The condition was first described clinically in 1938. The absence of

Barr body, consistent with the presence of one X chromosome, was noted in 1954 and cytogenetic confirmation was forthcoming in 1959. This and 45, XX or XY,-22 are the only non-mosaic, viable monosomies recorded in human beings; indicating the severe consequences of monosomy of all but the two smallest autosomes and a sex chromosome. However, individuals with Turner syndrome have about normal intelligence but underdeveloped ovaries, abnormal jaws, webbed necks and shield like chests. Congenital heart disease is also common, particularly preductal coarctation of the aorta and bicuspid aortic valve. Cardiovascular abnormalities are the single most important cause of increased mortality in children with Turner syndrome.

Further, Turner syndrome is the single most important cause of primary amenorrhea, accounting for one-third of the cases. For reasons not clear, approximately 50% of patients develop auto-antibodies directed to the thyroid gland and up to half of these develop clinically manifest hypothyroidism. Equally mysterious is the presence of glucose intolerance, obesity, and insulin resistance in a minority of patients.

18

The molecular pathogenesis is not completely understood. Both X- chromosomes are active during oogenesis and are essential for normal development of the ovaries. In Turner syndrome, fetal ovaries develop normally early in embryogenesis, but the absence of the second X- chromosome leads to an accelerated loss of oocytes, which is completed by age 2 years. In a sense, therefore, menopause occurs before menarche and the ovaries are reduced to atrophic fibrous strands, devoid of ova and follicles.

Because patients with Turner syndrome also have other abnormalities, it follows that some genes for normal growth and development of somatic tissues must also reside on the X-chromosome. Among the genes involved in Turner phenotype is the short stature homebox (SHOX) gene at Xp22.33

b) **Trisomy:** The presence of an extra chromosome is referred to as trisomy. The various trisomies are: Down syndrome (trisomy 21), Edward Syndrome (trisomy 18), and Patau syndrome (trisomy 13).

Down syndrome (Trisomy 21): Down syndrome is often called Trisomy 21 because most people with this condition have three copies of the number 21 chromosome-one of the smallest of the human autosomes. The Physician *John Langdon Down* first described this syndrome in 1866. Down syndrome was the first syndrome to be due to a chromosomal disorder, discovered by *Jerome Lejeune*. It affects about one in seven hundred live births. The most common finding in the newborn period is severe hypotonia. Usually the facial characteristic of upward sloping palpebral fissures, small ears and protruding tongue prompt rapid suspicion of the diagnosis. Most affected individuals are mildly to moderately mentally retarded and have congenital heart defects and a very high risk of acute leukemia (1/100). They are usually short and have a broad, short skull; hyperflexibilty of joints; and excess skin on the back of the neck.

An interesting aspect of this syndrome is the increased incidence among children of older mothers. Since the future ova are in the prophase I of meiosis since before birth, all ova are the same ages as the female. Presumably, older ova have an increased likelihood of non-disjunction of chromosome 21.

19

Recently, techniques of molecular genetics have been used to identify the origin of the three copies of chromosome 21 in large samples of individuals with Down syndrome.

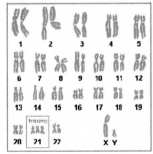

As expected, the overwhelming majority of the extra copies of chromosome 21 (95%) were of maternal origin and 5% were of mitotic origin, occurring either in the gonad of one of the parents or possibly post-zygotically in the fetus. Robertsonian translocations accounts for 4% of all cases and in roughly one-third of cases, parent is found to be carrier. Children with mosaicism are often less severely affected than those with full syndrome.

Edward syndrome (Trisomy 18): It affects one in ten thousand live births. Most affected individuals are females, with 80%-90% mortality by two years of age. The affected usually have an elfin appearance with small nose and mouth, a receding lower jaw, abnormal ears and lack of distal flexion creases on the fingers. There is limited motion of

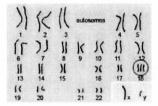

the distal joints and a characteristic posturing of the fingers, in which the little and index fingers overlap the middle two. The syndrome is usually accompanied by severe mental retardation.

Patau Syndrome (Trisomy 13): It affects one in twenty thousand live births. Diagnostic features are cleft palate, cleft lip, congenital heart defects, polydactyly, and severe mental retardation. Amorality is very high in the first year of life.

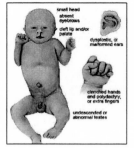

Other autosomal trisomies are known but are extremely rare. These include trisomy 8 (47,XX or XY,+8) and cat's eye syndrome, a trisomy of unknown, small acrocentric chromosome (47,XX or XY,{+ acrocentric}).

20

Chromosomal analysis usually reveals straightforward trisomy. Both disorders occur more frequently with advance maternal age, the additional chromosome being of maternal origin. Approximately 10% cases are caused by mosaicism or unbalanced re-arrangements particularly Robertsonian translocation in Patau syndrome.

Numerical abnormalities of sex chromosome: These are fairly common and cause less severe defects than autosomal abnormalities.

a) Klinefelter's Syndrome: It is one of the sex chromosome trisomy. The condition was first described by *Harry Klinefelter* in 1942. This karyotype is indicative of Klinefelter's syndrome because it has three sex chromosomes-a single Y chromosome and two X chromosomes, instead of the usual two *(47,XXY).* It presents a peculiar situation in which an individual with male phenotype is X-chromatin positive.

Patients are tall, thin, eunuchoid. They have long legs and poorly developed secondary sexual characters. Testes are smaller in size, the scrotum and penis may show hypoplasia. There is associated gynaecomastia. Pubic, chin, chest and axillary hairs are absent or poorly developed.

Molecular studies have shown that there is roughly equal chance that this will have been inherited from the mother or the father. The maternally derived cases are associated with advanced maternal age. A small proportion of cases show mosaicism e.g. (46,XY/ 47,XXY)

b) XXX Females: Birth surveys have shown that approximately 0.1 % of all females have a 47,XXX karyotype. These women have no physical abnormalities but can show a mild reduction in intellectual skills and sometimes quite oppositional behavior. This additional X chromosome is of maternal origin in 95% of cases and usually arises from an error in meiosis I.

c) XYY Males: This condition shows incidence of about 1:1000 in males in newborn surveys. Most 47, XYY men do not have any learning difficulties, although they can show emotional maturity and impulsive behavior. Physical appearance is normal and stature is usually above average. Intelligence is mildly impaired. The additional Y chromosome must arise either as a result of non-disjunction in maternal meiosis II or as a post-zygotic event.

B.   *Different cell lines (Mixoploidy):*

1. **Mosaicism:** It is defined as presence in an individual or in a tissue, two or more cell lines that differ in their genetic constitution but are derived from a single zygote. Chromosome mosaicism usually results from non-disjunction in an early embryonic mitotic division with the persistence of more than one cell line.

It is observed in Turner's syndrome and Down syndrome and the phenotype is less severe than in cases with complete enuploidy. Mosaicism has been documented for many other numerical or structural chromosomal abnormalities that could be lethal in non-mosaic form.

The clinical importance of chromosomal mosaicism detected prenatally may be difficult to assess. The abnormal karyotype detected by amniocentesis or chorionic villus sampling may be confined to placental cells, but even when present in the fetus, the severity with which the fetus will be affected is difficult to predict.

The single gene mutations occurring in somatic cells also result in mosaicism. In Mendelian disorders, this may present as a patchy phenotype, as in segmental neurofibromatosis type I. Germ line mosaicism is one explanation for the transmission of a genetic disorder to more than one offspring by apparently normal parents.

2.   **Chimerism**: It is defined as the presence in an individual two or more genetically distinct cell lines derived from more than one zygote. Human chimeras are of two types: Dispermic and Blood chimeras

A. ***Dispermic chimeras***: It results from double fertilization where by two genetically different sperm fertilize two ova and the resulting two zygote fuse to form one embryo. If the two zygotes are of different sex, chimeric embryo can develop in to an individual with true hermaphroditism and an XX / XY karyotyping.

B. ***Blood chimeras:*** It results from exchange of cells via placenta between non identical twins in-utero.

The concept of ***multifactorial or polygenic inheritance*** implies that a disease is caused by interaction of several adverse genetic and environmental factors. Unraveling the molecular genetics of the complex multifactorial diseases is much more difficult than for single gene disorders. Nevertheless, this is an important task, as these diseases account for the great majority of morbidity and mortality in developed countries. Example of one such disease with multifactorial or polygenic inheritance is neural birth defect.

Neural birth defects (NTDs), such as spina bifida and anencephaly, illustrate many of the underlying principles of multifactorial inheritance and emphasize the importance of trying to identify possible adverse environmental factors. These conditions result from defective closure of the developing neural tube during the first month of embryonic life. A defect occurring at the upper end of the developing neural tube results in either

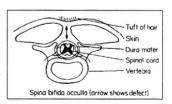

Spina bifida occulta (arrow shows defect)

exencephaly/anencephaly or an encephalocele. A defect occurring at the lower end of the neural tube results in a spinal lesion such as lumbrosacral myelocele or meningomyelocele, and a defect involving the head plus cervical and thoracic spine leads to craniorachischisis.

Anencephaly and craniorachischisis are not compatible with survival more than a few hours after birth. As with many malformations, NTDs can be classified etiologically under the headings of chromosomal, syndromal and isolated. Chromosomal causes include trisomy 13 and trisomy 18, in both of which NTDs show an incidence of around 5% to 10%. Syndromal causes include the relatively rare autosomal recessive disorder Meckel-Gruber syndrome. However, most NTDs represent isolated malformations in otherwise normal infants and appear to show multifactorial inheritance. Environmental factors include poor socio-economic status, multiparity and valproic acid embryopathy.

Geneticists believe that certain genes may play a role in damage to the neural tube, but the mother's diet during pregnancy also plays a role. A woman's risk of giving birth to an infant with a neural tube defect significantly decreases if she consumes adequate amounts of folic acid, a vitamin in the B complex, during the first three months of pregnancy and one month before conception.

Some common diseases that run in families but do not display an obvious pattern of inheritance are also thought to be multifactorial. Two examples are coronary heart disease and diabetes mellitus. In both cases, genes may cause a person to be predisposed to develop the disease, but lifestyle choices can help to prevent the disease from developing or from worsening after it occurs.

Diseases due to multifactorial Inheritance have the following important features:

1. The risk of expressing a multifactorial disorder is conditioned by the number of mutant genes inherited. Thus the risk is greater in siblings of patients having severe expression of the disorder. For example, the risk of cleft lip in the siblings of an index case is 2.5% if the cleft lip is unilateral but 6% if it is bilateral. Similarly, the greater the number of affected relatives, the highest is the risk for other relatives.

2. The rate of reoccurrence of the disorder is same for all first-degree relatives of the affected individual. Thus, if parents have had one affected child, the risk that the next child will be affected is between 2% to 7%. Similarly, there is the same chance that one of the parents will be affected.

3. Discrete phenotypes are difficult to recognize and a continuous variation in "susceptibility" exemplifies the typical situation.

4. The likelihood that both identical twins will be affected is significantly less than 100% but is much greater than the chance that both non-identical twins will be affected.

5. The risk of recurrence of the phenotypic abnormality in subsequent pregnancies depends upon the outcome in previous pregnancies. When one chl is affected, there is upto a 7% chance that the next child will be affected, but after two affected siblings, the risk rises to about 9%.

6. Expression of multifactorial trait may be continuous or discontinuous. In case of latter, disease is expressed only when the combined influences of the genes and environment cross a certain threshold.

Assigning a disease to this mode of inheritance must be done with caution. It depends on many factors but first on familial clustering and the exclusion of Mendelian and chromosomal modes of transmission. A range of levels of severity of a disease is suggestive of multifactorial inheritance, but variable expressivity and reduced penetrance of single mutant genes may also account for this phenomenon. Because of these problems, sometimes it is difficult to distinguish between Mendelian and multifactorial inheritance.

Isolated malformations that show multifactorial inheritance:

➢ Atrial Septal Defect
➢ Tetralogy of Fallot
➢ Patent Ductus Arteriosus
➢ Ventricular Septal Defect
➢ Hypospadias
➢ Renal agenesis, Renal dysgenesis
➢ Cleft lip/ cleft palate or both
➢ Congenital dislocation of hips
➢ Talipes
➢ Pyloric stenosis
➢ Gout

4. MITOCHONDRIAL DISORDERS

Not all DNA resides within the cell nucleus. Mitochondria have their own DNA consisting of double stranded circular molecule. It consists of 16567 base pairs that constitute 37 genes. The mitochondrial genome encodes 22 types of transfer and ribosomal RNA molecules that are involved in mitochondrial protein synthesis, as well as 13 of the polypeptides involved in respiratory chain system. Diseases affecting mitochondrial function may therefore be controlled by nuclear gene mutation and follow Mendelian inheritance, or may result from mutations within the mitochondrial DNA.

Both sperm and egg contain mitochondria, but at fertilization, a sperm contributes only the genetic material in its nucleus to the new life form. All of a person's mitochondria are genetic descendents of those mitochondria that were present in the egg before fertilization. *Therefore, mitochondrial disorders are transmitted solely through the mother.* Both males and females can be affected, but an affected male will not pass on the disorder to his children.

Conditions involving mitochondrial inheritance are rare, and they have been recognized only since the 1980s. One example is *Leber's hereditary optic neuropathy*, a cytoplasmically inherited disease. It was first described by Douglas Wallace and his colleagues in 1988. This is the first human disease traced to a specific mitochondrial DNA mutation.

The disease causes blindness with a median age of onset of 20-24 years. The onset age and phenotype are variable, depending upon the degree of heteroplasmy in the individual. Apparently, defects in mitochondria are not tolerable in the optic nerve, having great energy demand. It also does some damage to the heart. It was determined through pedigrees that the disease was transmitted only maternally. Sequencing of mitochondrial DNAs in affected families resulted in pinning down the disease to point mutation, a change of nucleotide 11778, which is in the gene for NADH dehydrogenase subunit 4. A guanine is changed to an adenine at codon 340 that converts an arginine to a histidine.

Because multiple copies of mitochondrial DNA are present in the cell, mitochondrial mutations are often heteroplasmic-that is a single cell will contain a mixture of mutant and wild type of mitochondrial DNA. With successive cell divisions, some cells will remain heteroplasmic but others may drift towards homoplasmy for the mutant or wild-type DNA. Large deletions, which make the remaining mitochondrial DNA shorter, may have a selective advantage in terms of replication efficiency, so that the mutant genome accumulates preferentially. The severity of disease caused by mitochondrial mutations depends on the relative proportions of mutant and wild type DNA present, but is difficult to predict in a given subject.

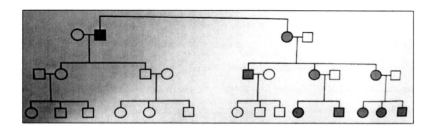

Pedigree of Leber's Hereditary Optic Neuropathy
(All progeny of an affected male are normal, but all children, male and female, of the affected female manifest disease)

Other disorders affecting mitochondrial function are:
1.   Myoclonic epilepsy and ragged red fibre disease (MERRF)
2.   Mitochondrial Encephalomyopathy, Lactic acidosis, and stroke like episodes (MELAS)
3.   Neurodegeneration, ataxia and retinitis pigmentosa (NARP)
4.   Leigh disease
5.   Barth syndrome
6.   Disorders of mitochondrial fatty-acid oxidation: a) Medium chain acyl- CoA Dehydrogenase deficiency; b) Long-chain and short chain acyl-CoA and long chain 3-hydroxyacyl-CoA Dehyrogenase deficiencies, c) Glutaric acidurias.

27

Genetic counseling dilemmas in mitochondrial diseases:

1. Some disorders of mitochondrial function are due to nuclear gene mutation
2. Many disorders caused by mitochondrial mutations are sporadic
3. It is not known whether the degree of heteroplasmy in the mother determines risk to offspring
4. Severity is very variable and difficult to predict
5. It is difficult to advise asymptomatic relatives who carry the mitochondrial mutation

III.   DIAGNOSIS OF GENETIC DISORDERS:

Diagnosis of genetic disorders requires examination of genetic material (chromosomes and genes). Hence two general methods employed are cytogenetic analysis and molecular analysis. Cytogenetic analysis requires karyotyping.

Normal Karyotype:

Human somatic cells contain 46 chromosomes; these comprise 22 homologous pairs of autosomes and two sex chromosomes, XX in female and XY in male. The study of chromosomes-karyotyping: is the basic tool of the cytogeneticist. The usual procedure of producing a chromosome arrest is to arrest mitosis in dividing cells in metaphase by the use of mitotic spindle inhibitors and then to stain the chromosomes. In a metaphase spread, the individual chromosomes take the form of two chromatids connected at the centromere.

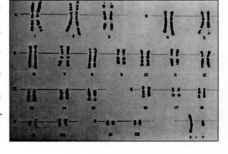

A karyotype is a standard arrangement of a photographed or imaged stained metaphase spread in which chromosome pairs are arranged in order of decreasing length. A variety of staining methods that allows identification of each individual chromosome on the basis of a distinctive and reliable pattern of alternating light and dark bands along the length of the chromosome have been developed. The one most commonly employed uses a Giemsa stain and is hence called G-banding. With G banding, approximately 400-800 bands per haploid set can be detected. The use of banding technique permits certain identification of each chromosome as well as delineation of precise breakpoints and other subtle alterations.

Prenatal chromosomal analysis: It should be offered to al the parents who are at the risk of cytogenetically abnormal progeny. It can be performed on cells obtained by amniocentesis, on chorionic villus biopsy or on umbilical cord blood. Some important indications are as follow:

✓   Advanced maternal age (>34 years) because of greater risk of trisomies.

✓   A parent who is carrier of a balanced reciprocal translocation, robertsonian translocation, or inversion.

✓   A parent with a previous child with a chromosomal abnormality.

✓   A parent who is a carrier of an X-linked genetic disorder.

Postnatal chromosomal analysis: It is usually performed on peripheral blood lymphocytes. Indications are as follow:

- Multiple congenital anomalies
- Unexplained mental retardation or development delay
- Suspected aneuploidy (e.g. features of Down syndrome)
- Suspected unbalanced autosome (e.g Prader-Willi syndrome)
- Suspected sex chromosomal abnormality
- Suspected fragile X syndrome
- Infertility
- Multiple spontaneous abortions

Many genetic disorders are caused by subtle changes in individual genes that cannot be detected by karyotyping. Traditionally the diagnosis of single-gene disorders has depended on the identification of abnormal gene products (e,g. mutant hemoglobin or enzymes) or their clinical effects, such as anemia or mental retardation (e.g. phenylketonuria).

It is now possible to identify mutations at the level of DNA and offer gene diagnosis for several mendelian disorders. The use of recombinant DNA technology for the diagnosis of inherited diseases has several distinct advantages over other techniques:

➢   It is remarkable sensitive. The amount of DNA required for diagnosis by molecular hybridization method can be readily obtained by 100,000 cells. Furthermore, the use of PCR allows several million fold amplification of DNA or RNA, making it possible to use as few as 100 cells or 1 cell for analysis.

➢   DNA based tests are not dependent on a gene product that may be produced only in certain specialized cells or expression of a gene that may occur later in life. Because virtually all cells of the body of an affected individual contain the same DNA, each post-zygotic cell carries the mutant gene.

There are two distinct approaches to the diagnosis of single-gene diseases by recombinant DNA technology: direct detection of mutations and indirect detection based on linkage of the disease gene with a harmless "marker gene."

DIRECT GENE DIAGNOSIS:

McKusick, an eminent geneticist, has appropriately called direct gene diagnosis the diagnostic biopsy of the human genome. Such diagnosis depends on the detection of an important qualitative change in the DNA. There are several methods of direct gene diagnosis, almost all based on PCR analysis, which involves exponential amplification of DNA from small quantities of starting material. If RNA is used as a substrate, it is first reverse transcribed to obtain cDNA and then amplified by PCR. This method is often abbreviated as RT-PCR.

•   One technique relies on the fact that some mutations alter or destroy certain restriction sites on DNA; this occurs in the gene encoding factor V. This protein is involved in the coagulation pathway, and a mutation affecting the factor V gene is the most common cause of inherited predisposition to thrombosis. Exon 10 of the factor

V gene and the adjacent intron have two Mnl1 restriction sites. A G-to-A mutation within the exon destroys one of the two Mnl1 sites.

To detect the mutant gene, two primers that bind to the 3' and 5' prime ends of the normal sequence are designed. By using appropriate DNA polymerases and thermal cycling, the DNA between the primers is greatly amplified, producing millions of copies of the DNA between the two primer sites. The amplified normal DNA and patient's DNA are then digested with the Mnl1 enzyme. Under these conditions, the normal DNA yields three fragments (67 base pairs, 37 base pairs, and 163 base pairs long); by contrast, the patient's DNA yields only two products, an abnormal fragment that is 200 base pairs and a normal fragment that is 67 base pairs long. These DNA fragments can be readily resolved by polyacrylamide gel electrophoresis and then visualized after staining with ethidium bromide under ultraviolet light.

• Mutations that affect the length of DNA (e.g., deletions or expansions) can also be detected by PCR analysis. Several diseases, such as the fragile-X syndrome, are associated with trinucleotide repeats. Two primers that flank the region affected by trinucleotide repeats are used to amplify the intervening sequences. Because there are large differences in the number of repeats, the size of the PCR products obtained from the DNA of normal individuals, or those with premutation, is quite different. These size differences are revealed by differential migration of the amplified DNA products on a gel. Currently the full mutation cannot be detected by PCR analysis because the affected segment of DNA is too large for conventional PCR. In such cases, a Southern blot analysis of genomic DNA has to be performed.

• A variety of PCR-based technologies that use fluorophore indicators to detect the presence or absence of mutations in "real time" (i.e., during the exponential phase of DNA amplification) have become available. This has significantly reduced the time required for mutation detection by removing the restriction digestion and electrophoresis steps used in conventional PCR assays. One example of high-throughput mutation analysis is the molecular beacon technology. Molecular beacons are hairpin-shaped fluorescent oligonucleotide probes that fluoresce only on hybridization to target sequences (wild-type DNA). In the presence of nucleotide mismatch because of mutations, effective pairing does not occur and there is no fluorescence.

INDIRECT DNA DIAGNOSIS: LINKAGE ANALYSIS

Direct gene diagnosis is possible only if the mutant gene and its normal counterpart have been identified and cloned and their nucleotide sequences are known. In a large number of genetic diseases, including some that are relatively common, information about the gene sequence is lacking.

Therefore, alternative strategies must be employed to track the mutant gene on the basis of its linkage to detectable genetic markers. In essence, one has to determine whether a given fetus or family member has inherited the same relevant chromosomal region(s) as a previously affected family member. It follows therefore that the success of such a strategy depends on the ability to distinguish the chromosome that carries the mutation from its normal homologous counterpart. This is accomplished by exploiting naturally occurring variations or polymorphisms in DNA sequences. Such polymorphisms can be grouped into two general categories: site polymorphisms and length polymorphisms.

- *Site polymorphisms* are also called *restriction fragment length polymorphisms (RFLPs)*. Examination of DNA from any two persons reveals variations in the DNA sequences involving approximately one nucleotide in every 200 to 500 base pair stretches. Most of these variations occur in non-coding regions of the DNA and are hence phenotypically silent; however, these single base pair changes may abolish or create recognition sites for restriction enzymes, thereby altering the length of DNA fragments produced after digestion with certain restriction enzymes. Using appropriate DNA probes that hybridize with sequences in the vicinity of the polymorphic sites, it is possible to detect the DNA fragments of different lengths by Southern blot analysis.

To summarize, *RFLP* refers to variation in fragment length between individuals that results from DNA sequence polymorphisms.

- *Length polymorphisms:* Human DNA contains short repetitive sequences of noncoding DNA. Because the number of repeats affecting such sequences varies greatly between different individuals, the resulting length polymorphisms are quite useful for linkage analysis. These polymorphisms are often subdivided on the basis of their length into microsatellite repeats and minisatellite repeats. Microsatellites are usually less than 1 kb and are characterized by a repeat size of 2 to 6 base pairs. Minisatellite repeats, by comparison, are larger (1 to 3 kb), and the repeat motif is usually 15 to 70 base pairs. It is important to note that the number of repeats, both in microsatellites and minisatellites, is extremely variable within a given population, and hence these stretches of DNA can be used quite effectively to distinguish different chromosomes. Microsatellites have assumed great importance in linkage studies and hence in the development of the human genome map. Currently, linkage to all human chromosomes can be identified by microsatellite polymorphisms

Single nucleotide polymorphisms (SNP) are a form of site polymorphism. As mentioned earlier, SNPs are the most common forms of polymorphisms in the human genome. They are found throughout the genome (e.g., in exons, introns, and regulatory sequences). SNPs serve both as a physical landmark within the genome and as a genetic marker whose transmission can be followed from parent to child. Because of their prevalence in the human genome and their stability, SNPs can be used in linkage analysis for identifying haplotypes associated with diseases, leading to gene discovery and mapping. In the last decade, SNPs have become the genetic marker of choice for the study for complex genetic traits.

Population studies have found associations between specific SNPs and multifactorial diseases such as hypertension, heart disease, or diabetes. For example, certain polymorphisms within the *angiotensinogen* gene are associated with variations in resting blood pressures and a predisposition to hypertension. A move is under consideration to map all SNPs in the human genome, which would facilitate the eventual construction of "SNP chips" for genetic risk profiling of individuals.

Because in linkage studies the mutant gene itself is not identified, certain limitations listed below become apparent:

1. For diagnosis, several relevant family members must be available for testing. With an autosomal recessive disease, for example, a DNA sample from a previously affected child is necessary to determine the polymorphism pattern that is associated with the homozygous genotype.

2. Key family members must be heterozygous for the polymorphism (i.e., the two homologous chromosomes must be distinguishable for the polymorphic site). Because there can be only two variations of restriction sites (i.e., presence or absence of the restriction site), this is an important limitation of RFLPs. Microsatellite polymorphisms have multiple alleles and hence much greater chances of heterozygosity. These are therefore much more useful than restriction site polymorphism.

3. Normal exchange of chromosomal material between homologous chromosomes (recombination) during gametogenesis may lead to "separation" of the mutant gene from the polymorphism pattern with which it had been previously coinherited. This may lead to an erroneous genetic prediction in a subsequent pregnancy. Obviously the closer the linkage, the lower the degree of recombination and the lower the risk of a false test.

Molecular diagnosis by linkage analysis has been useful in the antenatal or presymptomatic diagnosis of disorders such as Huntington disease, cystic fibrosis, and adult polycystic kidney disease. In general, when a disease gene is identified and cloned, direct gene diagnosis becomes the method of choice. If the disease is caused by several different mutations in a given gene (e.g., fibrillin-1; see earlier), however, direct gene diagnosis is not feasible, and linkage analysis remains the preferred method.

IV. GENETIC SCREENING:

Clinical geneticists and other health professionals use several screening tests and procedures to determine whether a person has a genetic disorder or is at risk of having a child with a disorder. These tests may be performed at various times in a person's life. Some genetic screening tests are routinely performed on newborns. Among adults, genetic screening is always voluntary.

A. Preimplantation diagnosis: A test that can be performed at the earliest possible stage of life is called pre-implantation diagnosis. This test is used in conjunction with in vitro fertilization, a procedure for uniting an egg and sperm in a laboratory rather than in a woman's body. Before an embryo created using in vitro fertilization is surgically implanted into the mother's uterus, physicians remove a cell from the developing embryo and analyze its DNA to learn if abnormalities associated with a specific genetic disorder are present. Although in vitro fertilization is a standard medical practice, removing cells from a developing embryo and preimplantation diagnosis are considered experimental procedures.

B. Prenatal Screening and Prenatal Testing:

These two types of medical tests may be used early in a woman's pregnancy to determine if her fetus has a defective gene or a chromosomal abnormality. Both procedures remove cells surrounding the developing fetus. The cells obtained have the same genetic makeup as the fetus and can be tested for genetic abnormalities.

In **chorionic villus** sampling, a doctor removes tissue from the chorionic villi, fingerlike projections that are part of the developing placenta, between 10 and 12 weeks of pregnancy. Using ultrasound guidance, the doctor inserts either a needle through the woman's abdominal wall or a thin, hollow tube called a catheter through her cervix to reach the chorionic villi. The doctor suctions out cells using a syringe.

Amniocentesis is usually performed between 15 and 17 weeks of pregnancy. In this procedure, a doctor uses ultrasound guidance to insert a needle through the abdominal wall into the amniotic fluid surrounding the fetus. Cells from the amniotic fluid are removed using a syringe.

Both procedures pose a slight risk for the developing fetus, and health professionals recommend these tests only in cases in which a mother or father has a family history of a genetic disorder or a known risk for chromosomal abnormalities.

Prenatal screening-Genetic screening performed during a pregnancy is used to identify fetuses at risk for certain genetic disorders. Usually, a multiple marker screen analyzes a pregnant woman's blood for the presence of three substances-**alpha fetoprotein, estriol, and human chorionic gonadotropin** that may signal certain problems in the fetus. This test is a screening test to identify fetuses with an extra chromosome or fetuses with a neural tube defect.

Chorionic villus sampling is a prenatal screening test performed at about the tenth week of pregnancy. A thin hollow tube called a catheter is inserted through the vagina and cervix into the uterus and is used to withdraw small amounts of the chorionic villus, which is part of the developing placenta.

In some instances, a sample of the chorionic villus is obtained through a needle inserted through the abdomen. Doctors isolate fetal cells from the chorionic villus and analyze them in the laboratory to determine if certain genetic abnormalities are present.

Amniocentesis is a prenatal screening test that is offered primarily to women who are 35 years or older at the time of pregnancy. This test is performed between the 14th and 20th weeks of pregnancy. Doctors insert a thin needle through the abdomen and into a woman's uterus, away from the fetus, to remove a few tablespoons of amniotic fluid. This fluid contains fetal urine and fetal cells, which can be used to prepare a karyotype-a photographic image that depicts all of the embryo's chromosomes in a cell.

A karyotype reveals whether a fetus has extra chromosomes, missing chromosomes, or chromosomes that have attached to one another in unusual ways. The cells in the amniotic fluid can also be used to check for the presence of certain DNA mutations and to determine whether enzymes present in the fluid are characteristic of certain genetic disorders.

C. Newborn Screening:

Genetic screening of newborns is necessary to identify those genetic disorders that would harm an infant if not treated immediately.

Newborns with **sickle-cell anemia** are at risk of dying from severe infections; these infants are given antibiotics immediately after being diagnosed with this disease.

Newborns with **phenylketonuria** lack the enzyme needed to convert phenylalanine, an amino acid present in food, into a different amino acid called tyrosine. As a result, phenylalanine can build up to toxic levels in the bloodstream, resulting in severe mental retardation. For infants diagnosed with this disease, doctors prescribe a special diet that lacks phenylalanine to prevent this damaging buildup.

Similarly, infants with **galactosemia** require a diet that is low in the sugar galactose to prevent the buildup of this substance to levels that produce seizures, mental retardation, and early death. In the United States and Canada, hospitals commonly screen newborns for phenylketonuria and galactosemia. Screening for sickle-cell anemia is performed for all infants in the United States and for infants of parents from at-risk groups in Canada.

D. Carrier Screening:

Genetic screening detects carriers of genetic disorders, people who have a single copy of a mutated recessive gene but are otherwise healthy. These tests are usually intended to diagnose autosomal recessive disorders that are common in individuals of certain ethnic backgrounds. For example, people of Eastern European Jewish ancestry may be screened to see if they are carriers for **Tay-Sachs disease**, **cystic fibrosis,** and an inherited neurological disorder called **Canavan disease.** In the United States and Canada, African Americans are at high risk for developing sickle-cell anemia. A blood disorder called **beta thalassemia** is more common in individuals of Greek or

Italian ancestry, and **alpha thalassemia**, a related condition, is more common in persons of Southeast Asian and Chinese ancestry.

Carrier testing identifies couples at risk of having an affected child so that they can make informed decisions about having children. Many couples choose to have children even if both partners are known to carry the same recessive gene. In such instances, some people undergo prenatal genetic testing to learn if a fetus has a disorder and decide at that time if they want to terminate the pregnancy.

Others use prenatal genetic testing to learn in advance the health status of their child so that they can prepare for a specialized delivery or surgery, or other treatment the infant may need.

E. Family History Screening:

Family pedigrees trace specific genetic characteristics through three or more generations. Pedigrees such as this one (**Figure 9**), which depicts the inheritance of a gene associated with **haemophilia,** help genetic counselors to identify which individuals in a family are at risk of either inheriting a genetic disorder or being a carrier for a disorder.

A medical family history helps identify healthy individuals at risk of developing a genetic disorder themselves, or of having a child with a genetic condition. In obtaining a family history, a health professional asks questions about the health of family members over a span of three or more generations. The information is recorded as a graphic image that incorporates symbols, such as squares, circles, triangles, and diamonds, to present a shorthand record of the medical family history. This image, called a pedigree, can reveal the multigenerational pattern of a genetic disorder.

For example, a dominant disorder affects at least one family member in each generation, whereas a recessive disorder may cluster in a single generation.

V. TREATMENT FOR GENETIC DISORDERS:

Gene therapy may someday be able to cure hereditary diseases, such as hemophilia and cystic fibrosis, which are caused by missing or defective genes.

In one type of gene therapy, **genetically engineered viruses** are used to insert new, functioning genes into the cells of people who are unable to produce certain hormones or proteins necessary for the body to function normally.

Currently, there are no permanent cures for genetic disorders, but many treatments are available. A procedure called gene therapy is on the horizon; it may eventually provide permanent cures for at least some genetic disorders.

For a few genetic disorders caused by an enzyme malfunction, it is possible to replace the malfunctioning enzyme with a functioning enzyme. For example, **Gaucher disease** is an autosomal recessive disorder marked by a shortage of an enzyme called **glucocerebrosidase.**

People with one type of Gaucher disease develop progressive bone disease and an enlarged spleen. They can be treated with enzyme replacement therapy, in which they receive regular intravenous infusions of synthetic enzymes that carry out the functions of glucocerebrosidase.

Most genetic disorders are treated using more than one type of treatment, in keeping with their complex and varied symptoms. For example, children with cystic fibrosis usually take pancreatic enzymes to help digest food and inhale medicines that are formulated to break up mucus in air passages. Parents of these children regularly clap their hand on the child's chest and back to loosen mucus in the lungs.

In some instances, surgeons may perform a lung transplantation to save a patient's life.

People with sickle-cell anemia commonly require drugs to combat pain and anemia and to prevent infections. They may receive blood transfusions to increase the number of normal red blood cells in their bloodstream. Adults with severe sickle-cell anemia sometimes benefit from an anticancer drug called **hydroxyurea,** which reduces the frequency of cell sickling, and from erythropoietin, a hormone that stimulates red blood cell production.

Some people with severe sickle-cell anemia benefit from bone marrow transplants.

An experimental procedure called gene therapy may have the potential to cure several fatal genetic disorders. Instead of treating symptoms of a disorder, gene therapy alters the genetic makeup of certain cells.

Gene therapy was first used in 1990 to treat children with an autosomal recessive condition called **adenosine deaminase (ADA)** deficiency. In the absence of the enzyme adenosine deaminase, T lymphocytes, a type of immune system cell, cannot develop normally. Children with ADA lack the immunity to fight off infections and typically die within the first years of life.

In experiments using gene therapy, a genetically modified virus was used to carry a normal ADA gene to the patient's immune cells. The inserted ADA gene then programmed the cells to produce the missing ADA enzyme, which led to normal immune function in those cells.

Gene therapy has also produced promising results in treating a rare immunologic disorder called chronic granulomatous disease, and it is being investigated in the treatment of cystic fibrosis and hemophilia.

VI. REFERENCES

1. Alan Stevens, James Lowe Human histology, Second Edition, Mosby, 1997.

2. Arnold Sorsby, Clinical Genetics, Second Edition, Butterworth, 1973.

3. Carlos Junqueria L, Jose Carneiro et.al., Basic Histology, Seventh Edition Appletion & Lange, 1991.

4. Champe and Harvey's, Illustrated Reviews : Biochemistry 2nd Edition, Lippin Cott – Raven Publishers, 2002.

5. Chandramouli, Text Book of Physiology, 2nd Edition, Jaypee Brothers Medical Publishers (P) Ltd., New Delhi.

6. Chaudhuri, Concise Medical Physiology, Third Edition, New Central Book Agency (P) Ltd., Calcutta, 2000.

7. Chummy S. Sinnatamby, Last's Anatomy, Tenth Edition, Churchill Livingstone 2001.

8. Cotran, Kumar and Collins Robbin's Pathologic Basics of Disease, Sixth Edition, W.B. Saundev's Company, 2001.

9. Datta. A. K. Essentials of Medical Genetics, ARK Publication, Kolkata, 2002.

10. David H. Cormack, Ham's Histology, Ninth Edition, J.B. Lippin Cott Company, Philadelphia 1987.

11. Edwards / Boucheier et.al., Davidson's Principles and practice of Medicine, Seventeenth Editon. ELBS with Churchill Living Stone, 1995.

12. Eugene Braunwald, Anthony S. Fauci et.al., HARRISON'S Principles of Internal Medicine, Fifteenth Edition, McGraw Hill Medical Publishing Division, 2001.

13. Gangane, Human Genetics, Second Edition, B.I. Churchill Living Stone Pvt., Ltd., New Delhi.

14. Ganong, Review of Medical Physiology, 20th Edition, Lange Medical Books/McGraw – Hill Medical Publishing Division 2001.

15. George M. Malcinski and David Freifelder's "Essentials of Molecular Biology" – Third Edition, Jones and BartLett Publishers, London.

16. Guyton & Hall, Text book of Medical Physiology, Tenth Edition, W.B. Saunders Company, Pennsylvania, 2000.

17. Harsh Mohan, Text Book of Pathology, Fourth Edition, Jaypee Brothers Medical Publishers (P) Ltd., 2000.

18. Helen Kreuzer and Adrianne Massey's Recombinant DNA and Biotechnology, Second Edition ASM Press, Washington (2001).

19. Helen M Kingston's ABC OF CLILICAL GENETICS, Second Edition, BMJ Publishing Group, 1997.

20. Inderbir Singh, Text Book of Human Histology, Fourth Edition, Jaypee Brothers Medical Publishers (p) Ltd., New Delhi, 2002.

21. Kanagasuntheram R et.al., Text Book of Anatomy, Orient Longman Limited, Hyderabed 1996.

22. Kissane et.al., Anderson's Pathology, Eighth Edition, The C.V. Mosby Company, Missouri, 1985.

23. Lawrence H. Bannister et.al., Gray's Anatomy, Thirty Eighth Edition, Churchill Livingstone, 1995.

24. Lodish, Berk et.al., Molecular Cell Biology, Fourth Edition, W.H. Freeman and Company, U.S.A, 2000.

25. Luiz Carlos Junqueria, Joes Carneiro's Basic Histology Text & Atlas, Tenth Edition, Mc Graw-Hill Companies, 2003.

26. Muthaya N.M, Physiology, JJ Publications, 2000.

27. Neville Woolf, Pathology Basic and Systemic, W.B. Saunder's Company Ltd., Landon, 1998.

28. PAL G.P., Basis of Medical Genetics, AITBS Publishers, New Delhi, 2003.

29. Robert and Young's Emery's Elements of Medical Genetics, Tenth Edition, Churchill Livingstone, 1998.

30. Robert H. Tamarin, Principles of Genetics, Sixth Edition, International Edition.

31. Robert K. Murray, Daryl K. Granner et.al., Harper's Biochemistry, Twenty Fifth Edition, Appletion & Lange Stamford, Connecticut, 2000.

32.Robert M. Berne, Matthew N. Levy et.al. Physiology, Third Edition, Mosey Year Book 1993.

33.Roland Lesson, Thomas S. Lesson et.al., Text Book of Histology, W.B. Saunder's Company, Philadelphia, 1985.

34.Sarada Subramanyan et.al., Text Book of human Physiology, S.Chand & Company Ltd., New Delhi, 1996.

35.Walter, Talbot, Walter & Iseral General Pathology, Seventh Edition, Churchill Livingstone, 1996.

36.William Boyd, A Text Book of pathology, Structure and Function in Disease, Eighth Edition, Lea & Feblger, Philadelphia 1949.

37.Winter, Hickey and Fletchev, Instant Notes Genetics, Second Edition, Viva Books Private Limited, New Delhi 2003.

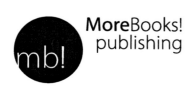
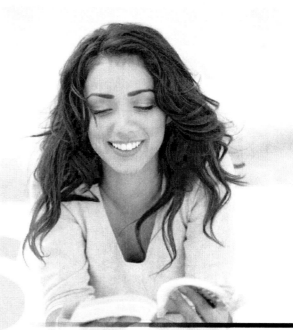

0 1341 1487999 9

CPSIA information can be obtained at www.ICGtesting.com
Printed in the USA
LVOW11s1725131115

462469LV00002B/444/P

9 783659 354953